ISBN: 978-0-9572777-2-4

First Published in the United Kingdom in 2011 by CMST

Produced by CMST

Dedication

This book is dedicated to my handsome son and my wonderful

family and friends

Contents

Introduction

My name is Jules Roberts and I am an experienced counsellor and behavioural coach, I also live with secondary breast cancer. I thought that I would put this short book together because facing a diagnosis of secondary breast cancer is a terrible shock; it is tough and has the potential to completely change your life forever.

If you are reading this book then I am guessing that you have either experienced that diagnosis or someone close to you has experienced it, so what can I tell you that you don't know already? In truth I may not be able to tell you anything or help you at all. This book is about what this disease can do to your mind, not about what the disease does to your body; I just want to share my experiences with you and the way that I have coped with them. I know that you can help yourself to cope with the terrors that you are facing, I know because I am. I have used some of the techniques that I have used with my clients and patients over the years, not necessarily clients who are experiencing cancer but individuals who are facing anxiety and anger issues, people who perhaps lack confidence or self-esteem. I will introduce you to what I call *'real time management'* and my (sometimes slightly warped) sense of humour.

Reading this book may have no effect on you at all or it may help you to work through your own thoughts and live the life that you love. I couldn't find a book to help me how to think about my diagnosis and I also know from my professional experience that not everyone wants to open up to strangers, even if they do appear in

the guise of experienced counsellors. So please read

through my ramblings and scribble your own thoughts

down too and I do hope that in some way it helps you

on your journey, even if that is just the short distraction

of the time that it takes you to flick through the book.

My Story

If you have read the introduction, you will already know that I am Jules Roberts, I am actually Julie but I consider that to be my *'Sunday name'*. I am in my late forties (2012) and back in 2009 I was diagnosed with breast cancer. I had a course of chemotherapy followed by surgery and then radiotherapy. My tumours are Her2 positive and so I also had the targeted therapy called Herceptin. This was part 1 of my personal cancer journey.

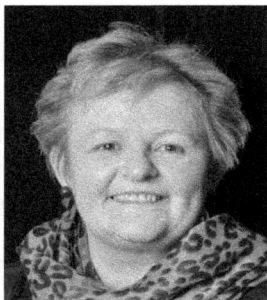

I have had lots of experience of living with cancer firstly I helped, as a teenager to, nurse my beloved nana Mabel. Nana Mabel had had breast cancer many years earlier and had enjoyed a long remission before succumbing to lung secondaries. At the age of fifty, my mum died, she too had breast cancer after previously surviving cervical cancer. Caring for my mum was hard work, she came to live with me and her condition demanded twenty four hour care. She was terrified of dying and her life and death had a marked effect on me during the following decade, and indeed on how I managed my own condition some sixteen years later.

Finally in 2004 my lovely partner, Steve Roberts was diagnosed with cancer in his kidney, he had a nephrectomy which initially appeared to be a great success but only twelve weeks later extensive bone secondaries were

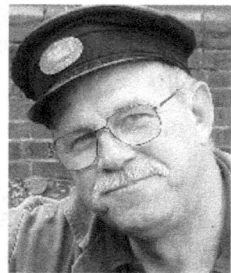

discovered but only after he had suffered a fracture of the vertebrae in his neck. From then on Steve was confined to a wheel chair and spent some considerable time in an orthopaedic halo. Amazingly he survived for eleven months and it was through sharing his journey that I learned so much about living with secondary cancer. I never thought that I would be in a similar situation so soon afterwards. Steve taught me so much about personal attitudes towards the condition, so called looking on the bright side of life and reframing your thoughts. He taught me more than several years of professional training had given to me. Let me explain.........

December 6th 2005 Steve was lying in a hospital bed. He had been to the operating theatre and had his orthopaedic halo fitted to stabilise the neck injury caused by his condition. The orthopaedic surgeon stopped by his bed on his ward round and a very depressed Steve bluntly asked him "I suppose that I am going to die of cancer now then am I?" and this marvellous surgeon said "well that is entirely up to you, dying of cancer is an option but most people prefer to live with it". After days of sadness and talk of funerals and flowers a new light switched on inside his mind. Instead of contemplating death and dying he would once again focus on life and living. He had been given permission to live!

Amazingly despite the broken neck Steve managed to walk again, only a few paces but he walked, he also drove his precious car again. We had a fantastic eleven months together and when he finally died, well it was the right time.

So as you can see I have lived 'with' cancer for most of my life, and learned so much from my nana, mum and partner. Now please don't get me wrong, as you and I both know losing a loved one is hell but living with them through their personal trials is a journey well-travelled. When I had my primary diagnosis I really thought that I knew how I would cope, I had been through it enough times, what I didn't know is that it would be so much easier, for me, but not necessarily for my family. It was so different. When Steve had been diagnosed I truly felt as though my world was falling apart. Not only was I concerned about myself and how I would cope with what was to come but I constantly worried about how

Steve felt. His emotional and physical needs were (in my mind) significantly greater than mine. I've heard people say that it's harder to be the partner than the patient but I'd never really felt the truth of it before. When I had my own diagnosis it was all about me, I didn't have to carry the weight of someone else's pain. And so for me my primary diagnosis was a thousand times easier than my partner's diagnosis. From here on, it [life] would be all about me and if that sounds selfish, then so be it.

On December 24th 2010 at 11:05 I was told that my cancer had spread into both my lungs and this is where this book begins.

24th December 2010

Warrington Hospital

I ran up the stairs to get my scan results because I quite simply did not have the time or the inclination to be bothered queuing for the lift, the breast clinic waiting area was standing room only. Fortunately I didn't have to wait too long before my turn, and I was in a bit of a hurry. It was Christmas Eve, phone calls to make, food to cook, wine to drink! My son was staying with me on Christmas Eve and then going off to stay with his pal who had just got himself a flat. I had promised to cook a Christmas lunch for them to share at the new gaff.

And then suddenly I had a storm in my head like the sea smashing against rocks, absolute chaos and no way of calming the seas or stilling the gales.

Tumours, both lungs, extensive, oncology, immediate, time, Christmas, just a barrage of words that I couldn't process. Now I don't know what it was like for you but for me, well I just wanted to go somewhere quiet and process my thoughts, and not a hope of that on Christmas Eve.

I have to admit it never crossed my mind that this news might upset other people and perhaps I should keep quiet until after the holiday. My family and friends always ask about my hospital appointments and when they did I just blurted it out, "it's come back, it is in both of my lungs and there is no cure". I was completely selfish but I was in a terrible state of shock.

I can't remember much more of either Christmas Eve or Christmas Day. I sent everyone away and went to the best thinking place in the world, my bed, except I couldn't think because the storm was still raging inside my head, the waves crashing against the rocks, completely out of control. I think that I probably spent the next thirty six hours watching back to back Midsomer Murders and Morse repeats.

When I got up on Boxing Day morning I really couldn't bear to be in the house for a moment longer than was absolutely necessary, so I packed my credit cards and I headed for the sales. What a catastrophe! My normal behaviour would be to find something that fits (I am a large lady) and buy one in every colour with shoes and accessories. The fact that six months later my purchase may end up in the charity shop has never been a relevant consideration. My new 'terminal' behaviour was to walk around trying things on, trousers, shoes, jackets and then quietly advise myself in my innermost conspiratorial voice, *"no point buying them, you won't wear them out"*. What tosh? I don't think that I had actually worn anything out since my school uniform. A new behaviour was emerging here, the behaviour of a doomed woman.

I can remember that day at the sales so vividly, colours, sounds feelings everything was heightened, my emotions were finely tuned and yet the storm kept crashing around inside my head relentlessly, too much, far too much, system going into overload. I headed home and went straight back to bed, I didn't even check my Facebook page, things were that dire.

Back in the relative safety of my own bed I could feel

the pain increasing, it was all around my ribs, my back and my shoulders the cancer must be growing fast, I didn't have any pain before Christmas and now every movement was complete agony. How many times in my life have I treated someone for anxiety with exactly those symptoms?

New Year's Eve saw me once again back at the hospital but this time at the CanTreat unit at Halton Hospital where I had had my previous treatments. The oncologist was very truthful with me, but not unkind. He said that he couldn't make me any promises or predictions and that I could start capecitabine (an oral chemotherapy drug) and Herceptin the following Friday.

I was now at an all-time low, his words translated inside my head to 'take your library books back, call at the florist and go home and wait', and still the storm crashed around inside my head. The wind was getting stronger and the waves higher and the sound of the sea lashing against the rocks was getting louder and louder. Straight back to bed and a date with D.I Barnaby, thank goodness for the Sky Plus series link feature. I am not sure how long I stayed there, a couple of days probably and at one point I remember lying rigid and still as if I was in a coffin to see if I could work out what it would be like to be dead. And then suddenly out of nowhere amongst the thrashing waves and the dangerous rocks I actually thought that I saw a small wooden boat and I thought "I have a choice to make here"

I could really panic lying here in a pretend coffin and that small boat would soon be drift wood, or I could take control. Calm the winds push back the tides and save that little wooden boat from destruction. For a moment I actually thought that I saw a ray of sunshine and then there was a little bit of clarity and I asked myself a very important question, "what has actually changed here?" And the waves stopped crashing against the rocks and the winds started to ease down, I watched the clouds scud across my inner landscape and as the sun broke through the clouds I realised that nothing much had actually changed since 11:05 on Christmas Eve.

☑ The cancer had returned………

  Well that was always going to be a possibility

☑ I was going to die

  I never actually signed up for immortality – death

is inevitable for all of us

☑ I needed more treatment

Well, yes that was a bit of a bummer, but chemotherapy had always been my friend

As suddenly as that my mind cleared and now I could make a plan. As a solution focussed counsellor and coach I decided that I should ask myself, "How would you treat a client?"

Begin with the End in Mind

When I begin the counselling process, I usually want to know where my client wants to be at the end of the process. After all I need to know what to work towards. Most clients know exactly what they don't want

"I don't want to live with him anymore"

"I hate my job; I just don't want to work there anymore"

"I don't want to feel like this"

Reframing the don't wants into do wants is a part of the process and so true to form I started a list of my don't wants

"Don't want to die"

"Don't want to be ill"

"Don't want to be with people that upset me"

"Don't want to waste my final weeks/months/years"

Okay so just like every other client I knew exactly what I didn't want. What don't **you** want? Writing a problem or issue down can be enormously therapeutic. It is a little bit like tipping it out of your head and on to the written page, in my type of work this is known as journaling. Writing things down allows you to clarify your thoughts and feelings, thereby gaining valuable self-knowledge. It's also a good problem-solving tool; oftentimes, you can thrash out a problem and come up with solutions more easily on paper. Journaling about traumatic events helps you to process them by fully exploring and releasing the emotions involved. I kept a journal all through my mum's illness and also through Steve's. I reckoned that it kept me sane, many would argue.

Make a 'Note to Self', what don't you want, write everything down, there is a space for your thoughts.

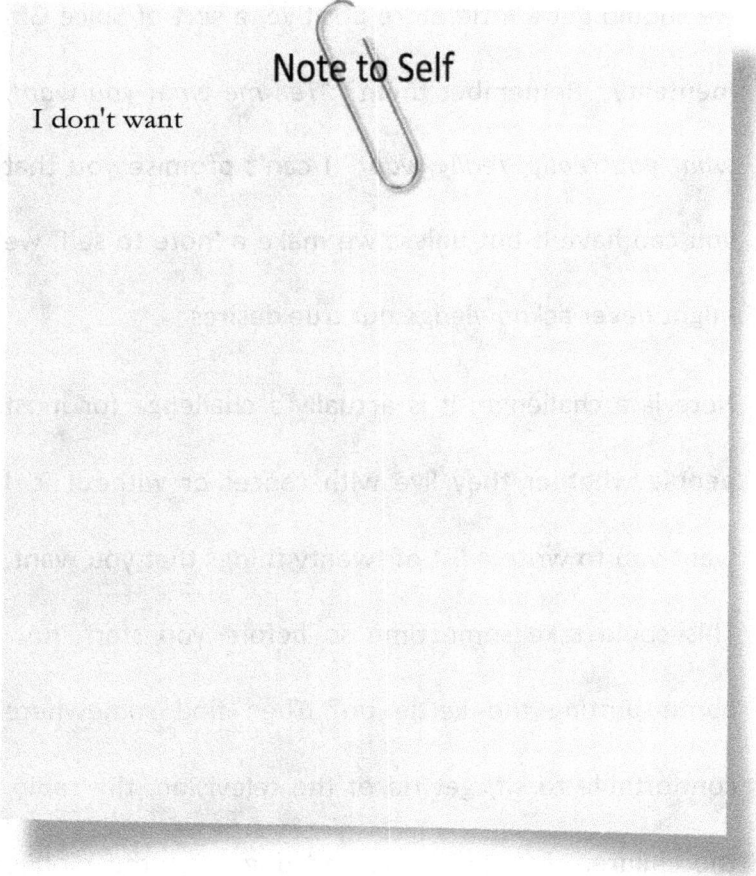

Note to Self

I don't want

Now that we have sorted what we don't want perhaps we should get a little more positive, a sort of Spice Girl mentality. Remember them? *"Tell me what you want, what you really, really want"* I can't promise you that you can have it but unless we make a 'note to self' we might never acknowledge our true desires

Here is a challenge; it is actually a challenge for most people whether they live with cancer or without it. I want you to write a list of twenty things that you want. This could take some time so before you start, how about putting the kettle on? Then find somewhere comfortable to sit, get rid of the television, the radio, the children, husband, cats and dog. Put the mobile phone in the fridge and just allow your mind to wander somewhere special where you can imagine or create

some wonderful ideas to put on your list

Note to Self

This is what I want, what I really, really want...

1)

2)

3)

4)

5)

6)

7)

8)

9)

10)

Note to Self

And it goes on, don't give up just keep writing

11)

12)

13)

14)

15)

16)

17)

18)

19)

20)

To think of twenty things that you want is really quite a task, and now that you have made your list I am going to ask you to pull it apart. Be like teacher now, red pen at the ready…………….

I want you to cross through with a red pen anything that is unrealistic or down right impossible, for example world peace or wanting to live forever. We are going to do some serious work with this list, so now I want you to re-write it but this time miss out the stuff that we have just crossed off and make the items on the list measurable. So for example if one of your list items is *'a big family holiday'* then I want to know where to and when by, so that may translate to *'a family trip to South End in May'*. When you have created a specific and measurable list I want you to prioritise it and we do that by re-writing it in the order that we want to do things or the things that are most important are top of the list. Take your time re-writing the list, it is important.

Note to Self

Actually this is what I want, what I really, really want...

1)

2)

3)

4)

5)

6)

7)

8)

9)

10)

Note to Self

Actually this is what I want, what I really, really want...

11)

12)

13)

14)

15)

16)

17)

18)

19)

20)

Some people call this a bucket list or a list of dreams.

Now that you have your list, you probably want to get

started upon it. Sorry, you can't! Not yet because there

is some serious stuff that you need to get out of the way

first.

Miracle Question

I often see clients who are quite stuck in a terrible rut, they really can't see the wood from the trees. They know what they don't want and haven't given too much thought to what they do want, all that they know is that they want something different, and so to give their mind a work out I ask them a 'miracle question' which goes something like this........

"Suppose that you went to bed tonight and whilst you were asleep a fairy godmother popped in, you don't know that she is there though because you are asleep. She will grant you a miracle but that miracle cannot be immortality. What will your life be like when you wake up in the morning?"

Go on, give it a go, you show me yours and I will show

you mine!

Note to Self

When I wake up in the morning I will…....

Note to Self

Jules's

I will wake up I the morning and all of the messy practical stuff will be sorted out so that my family aren't in a mess when I croak, and then I am just going to do the things that I want to do. I am going to enjoy every moment. AND if I realise that I am not enjoying myself then I will stop what I am doing and find something that I feel happier doing. I am going to be really, really grateful for every day that I have and I am going to be true to myself. From now on my life is all about me!

Fortunately I absolutely love my work and so I wasn't going to have to make many drastic changes but that said the changes that I do want to make can't happen until I have sorted out the practical stuff and 'got my house in order'. I know exactly what I need to do before I can really relax and get started with my 'bucket list'

The Practical Stuff

Step 1 – Money

☑ Check that to see if you are entitled to any benefits, the

easiest and least painful way to do this is to contact

Macmillan Cancer Support. You can find the benefits

information at

http://www.macmillan.org.uk/HowWeCanHelp/FinancialSupport/FinancialSuppo

rt.aspx   or you can telephone 0808 808 0000 (UK only)

☑ Now is the time to check the small print on any insurance

policies or mortgage protection policies. Some policies pay

out on serious illness. If so don't hesitate, you have paid

into them and now is the time to capitalise on them.

Step 2 – Work

If you don't work go straight to step 3

If you have been working up to this point you may want to review your priorities remember the list that we made? Will you have the time or the inclination to do all of this if you are still working? Perhaps you may want to consider reducing your hours or you may even decide to stop working all together. Personally I couldn't stand not to work; I love my job and want to continue for as long as possible. You will need to consider your financial situation and you may want to discuss your thoughts, feeling and ideas with your family and friends but before you do please complete the list on the next page, get those thoughts out of your head and on to the paper, it may well help you to see things much more clearly.

Work For	Work Against

I now know what I think so now for the biggie................
How do I feel about this?

Step 3 – Planning Your Funeral

If this is too much for you right now remember you don't have to do this. Not now and if you don't want to not ever, someone else will take care of it.

Now as you may be starting to realise my sense of humour can be a little bit warped and believe it or not I actually enjoyed doing all of this. Now don't get me wrong, I am not looking forward to it and I don't want it to happen any time soon. I do though want it to be my funeral, my goodbye and not someone else's well-meaning intentions.

I am guessing that you may find this difficult so I have devised a little tick list, just to get you going. This works as a starting point and if you don't do anything else in preparation at least your family or close ones will have a good idea of what you had in mind, so go on. Take a deep breath and tick the boxes. You can always tear this page out of the book and leave it with the person that you are closest to.

Funeral Plan Check List

Religious Service ☐	Or	Humanitarian Service ☐
Burial ☐	Or	Cremation ☐
Church ☐	Or	Straight to the crematorium ☐
Hymns ☐	Or	Songs ☐
My two favourite songs or hymns are		
Flowers ☐	Or	Donations ☐
Donations to:		
Mourning Dress ☐	Or	Bright and Beautiful ☐

STOP! Enough now, go and make a coffee (or a double gin and tonic!). This is a big step taken especially if you haven't even thought of it before.

Step 4 - Advanced Directive

Let me tell you a little story, I recently heard someone who is very close to me talking about a friend who is really quite poorly. A part of the conversation revolved around, what I should call for the sake of politeness, 'a toilet accident'. My pal said, "She must be horrified living like this, it makes you wish that euthanasia was legal doesn't it?"

Well I don't mind admitting to you that overhearing that little snippet got me a tad worried, probably unnecessarily, that the first time that I don't quite make it to the loo that I might be taken into the garden and shot at dawn! *(I always was the dramatic type)* and so I thought that I might need to make some inquiries about how to avoid such misunderstandings. I was born into the Christian tradition and to me life is life. Now I understand that you might not feel the same way as me but whatever your belief system the same preparation still applies. After a little bit of research or in more modern terms Googling, I discovered a marvellous organisation called Compassion in Dying, you can get much more information from their website, www.compassionindying.org.uk.

To put it in a nutshell for you, I have created what I call an Advanced Directive, although some people will call it a living will, or an Advanced Decision. An Advanced Decision is a document that allows you to set out your wishes and preferences for medical treatment in advance, in the event that you become unable to communicate with your health team (for example, if you fall into a coma or develop dementia). The refusal of medical treatment, including life-prolonging medical treatment, is legally binding with an Advance Decision. This organisation has a pack that you can download with a template in it so that you can create your own directive. I didn't use a template but I have utilised their ideas, all of my care team have a copy of my Advanced Directive as do my family and friends. I review and if necessary I update the directive once every three months. Whatever your belief system for end of life care you can ensure that your wishes are known and carried out as you would want them to be. There is loads of information on the website all of the information is completely free. This organisation is a charity and there is a page to give a donation should you want to. Compassion in Dying is the only charity that supports people to know and exercise their rights at the end of life.

Step 5 - Making a Will

You may be well organised and have a last will and testament prepared, many people don't even want to think about making a will in case it somehow speeds up a visit from the grim reaper!

Having a will is so important and will certainly be a great help to those you leave behind. Many families are quite complicated these days especially as divorce and remarriage are now very much the norm. If you want to be sure about your wishes it really is important to make that will. You may even be eligible to have your will prepared free of charge; Quality Solicitors is a national group of law firms that have outlets throughout the UK and they operate a scheme that provides eligible people to have their will prepared free of charge.

Details about making a will are available on the Quality

Solicitors website (www.qualitysolicitors.com) including your local branch.

Why make a Will?

If you die without making a Will you will be "intestate" and the law will automatically determine how your property is distributed and who administers your affairs after death.

This may not necessarily be in a way you would have wanted.

Executors:

At least one Executor must be appointed, but if your Will contains trusts or provisions for children under eighteen, at least two are required.

They can include, for example, a family member, a friend, (remember to ask them first) or a professional advisor, including Quality Solicitors. Professionals will charge for their services.

Guardians

The appointment of guardians in a Will can avoid disputes within the family and ensure your children will be brought up by those people you consider most appropriate for this important task.

Legacies

Do you want to give a specific legacy (a specified item to a specified person) or a pecuniary legacy (a gift of a specific amount of money to a specified person)

Once all liabilities and legacies have been paid who is to get the rest of your estate (the residue)?

You may also consider who will benefit instead should your first choice of beneficiary die before you.

Well that has given you plenty to think about hasn't it, probably time for a coffee now?

This information is provided in its complete form at

http://www.qualitysolicitors.com/alb/services/wills/

Step 6 – Hospital Appointments

Hate them, hate them, hate them!

During the last year or so I have been having regular chemotherapy and now a new targeted therapy called Lapatinib. I had to change from Herceptin because it didn't quite work for me. I have tried a few different chemotherapy drugs too; my tumours don't seem to want to respond to many treatments. I have had to see my Oncologist quite regularly and I really don't like doing that. Not that there is anything wrong with my oncologist, (although I did nick name him Lord Voldermort for a while there!) I just don't like the whole hospital thing, possibly because I don't often get good news and also when I am going to hospital I have to think about cancer whereas I don't normally think about it much at all. I refer to my condition as a 'cellular malfunction', so far I am not ill and absolutely refuse to allow anyone to suggest otherwise, unless it gets me benefits, like not washing up!

One of my luxuries is my Kindle (an eBook reader), now I love that baby! I enjoy reading and carrying a kindle is so much lighter than carrying around a raft of paperback books. My hospital preparation involves

☑ Writing a list of questions that I need answering

☑ Ensuring that I have plenty to read

☑ Packing a bottle of water

☑ Packing a small packet of tissues in case I need to cry

☑ Prepare short sleeved comfortable clothes that are easy to remove

With a predefined hospital routine I do not need to even think about hospitals until I am preparing to go there. Make a 'note to self'; what would make your hospital visits easier

Note to Self

My hospital appointments would be easier if.........

Step 7 – Tiredness

Wow, I didn't know that it was possible to feel so tired and yet remain awake. Tiredness is probably one of the most debilitating aspects of this condition.

Some nights I work quite late, until around 9:30pm, on these days I make sure that I have the mornings as 'my time'. If I am feeling really, really stiff and tired I will go for a swim, but you could do any type of exercise, walking, gym etc. I am under five feet tall and wear a good size twenty, and so you may deduce Dear Holmes, exercise has never been a priority, until NOW.

Summoning up the motivation to go to the swimming pool is the hardest part; I now make sure that my swim bag is always packed and ready so that when the fancy takes me I can just grab my bag and go. If I had to mess around getting shampoo and clean towels I would probably be demotivated before I had got out of the front door.

When I get back from my swimming session I still sometimes feel tired, sometimes more tired than when I went but it is a completely different sort of tired. You and I both know that some days are more tiring that others, and so it is probably best to be prepared to shorten your day, take regular breaks and please try the exercise route, I wish that I had done it years ago. What preparations can you make that will make exercising easier? Have a think about it and make a Note to Self

Note to Self

Exercise would be easier if.........

Step 8 - Friends (and the things that they say!)

Telling friends and family about your diagnosis can be quite traumatic, for them to hear and for you to have to say. Some people will take it better than others. I remember when I had my primary diagnosis one of my friends blurted our *"will you still be here for Christmas!"* I responded without really thinking *"why? Have you bought my present already?"* and *we both fell about laughing!* Unfortunately it doesn't always happen quite so easily, many of your friends and family may not know how to cope with your news.

I cannot tell you how to tell them, we are all unique individuals with our own use of language and dialect, what I can say though is it is probably best to keep it simple and to the point. Once you have given your news try and remain quiet for a second or two because the people that care about you will need time to process what you have just told them. There may be tears and hugs or disbelief and sometimes even anger. You may even experience encouragement, you would not believe the amount of times that I have heard someone say to me *"you can beat it"*. I told one of my friends of my predicament by simply saying *"my cancer has come back and now I am stuck with it forever"*

There really is no easy way of imparting this news, so go easy on yourself. No matter how many times that you have to say it it probably won't get any easier and you will elicit different reactions too. Perhaps you may want to formulate a simple sentence that flows easily and gets to the point, you know what I am going to say next don't you? Why not try writing something down ...., in fact if you find it hard to talk to your friends you could always write them a note or a card explaining the way that you feel.

Step 9 - Olive Branches and Hobnail Boots!

There may well be people in your life that you have lost contact with over the years or people that you have argued with and fallen out with, conversely there may be people in your life that you wish you had lost contact with. You may well find yourself thinking about the people that are not in your life now and wondering where they are. Thomas Jefferson once said

"never put off until tomorrow what you can do today",

and this has been my mantra if there is someone out there that you want back in your life, then today may well be the day to 'extend the olive branch'. Thinking about quotes I seem to remember reading somewhere that Mark Twain also said ...

"Never put off till tomorrow what you can do the day after tomorrow".

So perhaps you may just decide to save your energy after all and leave the past where it is? Only you can decide.

Step 10 - Being a Mum

I have heard cancer called many things, I have heard to cancer being referred to as a gift, and also I have heard cancer being referred to as a thief. And if there is any truth in either of those references then I am sure that collectively we will find them. I am a mum and cancer cannot ever stop me from being a mum. I may become less able or inclined to do the practical things that mum's do, but that does not stop me from actually being a mum. My son is an adult and he now has a child of his own, perhaps your children are also grown up or you may have young children who are still dependent upon you for everyday tasks. If your condition restricts your daily activity, then I am sure that you will be very frustrated with yourself. Being a mum is a bit like being a male or female, a Jew or a Christian, it isn't about what you do, it is about who you are, being too tired to make trifle or go horse-riding doesn't stop you from being a mum.

Experience has taught me to give children enough information that they need to understand what is happening around them so that they can feel secure, answer their questions in a way that they can understand. When they need more information they will ask for it. It is really important to choose your words carefully when talking to your children, saying things like 'passed away' or 'gone to sleep' can be very confusing using the right words, dying and death gives clarity to a young mind. I have found this philosophy of basic honesty to be very good advice over the years.

If you don't tell your children what is happening then they will soon start to feel insecure, they will instinctively know that something isn't right and may well worry that something that they have done has caused the problem.

If they can talk to you openly then they will trust you and support you, children often cope much better than we think that they will.

Frank A. Clark said

"There's nothing that can help you understand your beliefs more than trying to explain them to an inquisitive child"

Back to the List

I haven't forgotten about it, honest there are though just a few more things that I need to address first. These are things that I have done and you might think *"No way!"*, *"morbid"*, *"horrible"* and that is fine too, but I just wanted to share them with you, so deep breath and here goes.

I have had some professional photographs taken of my healthy self. I have done this because being a 'little fat bird' posing for photographs has never been my thing, but I remember desperately searching for photographs of my mum after she had died and the good ones were few and far between. Your family and friends will want a visual reminder of you; you don't necessarily need a professional photographer just make sure that you take camera with you when you go out. Record the moments of joy, fun and happiness, they are really important, oh, and if like me you have had loads of chemo…….. Make sure that you have got your lippy on. We don't want to scare the future generations do we?

I have written personal letters to the important people in my life to be distributed after my death, why have I done this? (*I can hear you thinking that from here you know!*)

☑ To me it seemed like the natural thing to do

☑ My death and probably the events leading up to it will have a lasting effect on my family and friends and I want them to know that I value them

☑ Because I am a bit of a control freak and want to have a 'voice' from beyond the grave

Now that was brutally honest and sometimes that is the only way to say it.

November the 7th 2011 saw the premature birth of my first grandchild. I hope that I have got a bit more life in me yet

but I don't know (nor ever will)
whether he will remember me and
so I have put together a hard back
book full of pictures and a brief

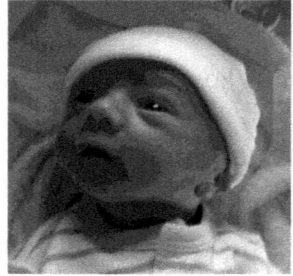

outline of my life. I have even included a little bit about those

who have gone before, remember my Nana Mabel, my mum

and partner Steve Roberts, they feature in the book too.

I cannot begin to tell you how many tears that I shed putting

the book together, I sobbed and sobbed and yet it was

surprisingly therapeutic. I have long been an advocate of

moving thoughts out of my head and on to paper and I would

advise you to give it a go. Just pick up a pencil and a note

book and write down thoughts as they pop up. No need to

read them back to yourself for a while, just write. The book

that I have prepared for my little grandchild is away in the safe along with the letters for the grownups, my funeral plan and a copy of my advanced directive.

Also in the Safe

Do you remember that miracle question? Where I wanted all of the messy practical stuff done so that I could enjoy every moment? Well this is where it all comes together and I can get back to the 'bucket list'. I bought a small safe to store all of my important stuff away. In addition to all of the things that we have discussed this far I have also made several lists that I have popped into the safe too, once again this is just to make things easier for those that are grieving .

My lists includes my computer passwords and

A list of all bank accounts, including

☑ Bank name

☑ Account number

☑ Sort code

☑ Pin

A list of all of my domestic and utility accounts with

☑ Account number

☑ Phone number

☑ Addresses

A notification list, this is a list of friends and family and acquaintances that may wish to be informed of my demise. The list includes

☑ Name

☑ Telephone Number

☑ Relationship, e.g work colleague, school friends.

These lists aren't too arduous and will help those that you have left behind. Perhaps there are other lists that you need to make that are relevant to your personal circumstances. Make a note to self of the type of lists that you need.

Note to Self

I need to write lists for

Real Time Management

I have always struggled with the concept of time, philosophically that is. Is time linear or some type of matrix, perhaps this is a discussion for another time? The idea of time travel has always fascinated me and I begged my son to call my new grandchild **T**omas **A**rchie **R**obert **D**avid **I**gnatius **S**tephen (by the way only two of my friends got that joke!)

Now all things being equal, time is very important to you and I, we are possibly to not going to achieve the coveted three score years and ten and so we must manage our time wisely. I don't know how you feel about time but I am guessing that you have given it some serious thought, and so I thought that I would share with you how I manage my time. Let's deal with time in these categories; it makes it easier to manage.

The Past – it has gone, it cannot be changed, although how we think about it can be changed. If you spend a lot of time here you will miss out on the here and now.

The Future – I have always been a planner and an organiser and lived very much in the future. On Easter Sunday 2006 I was sat at my desk writing my work schedules for the following week when I had a 'light bulb' moment. I simply glanced up and saw Steve sat on the sofa reading his newspaper and I suddenly realised that we would probably never have an Easter Sunday together again. I was deeply shocked and this moment of clarity had a marked effect upon me. I consciously started to live in the present, the here and now.

The Present – What do I mean by living in the present?

I quite simply mean concentrating on the here and now. If we are constantly looking backwards you cannot possibly focus on what is happening right now and totally engage with the present. If you fret about the future you cannot possibly focus on what is happening right now. Enjoying the here and now is your priority; it is all that we really have.

My greatest problem was living in the future and planning ahead in such detail that I wasn't enjoying the here and now. Whilst it is good to have plans and goals, once they have been decided (like the plans that we have made and put on the bucket list) our thoughts and experiences must come back to the here and now. This is the only time that we can live, the only time that we can actually experience because when all things are said and done, when we wake up in the morning we wake up in the here and now not in tomorrow.

When I wake up each morning I do a body audit, that simply means that I wiggle everything that is wiggleable and if it doesn't hurt then I thank my lucky stars that I have the here and now to enjoy. The fact that you and I live with cancer makes absolutely no difference, someone who doesn't live with cancer can still only experience now. Regardless of your state of health, your financial outlook or your IQ the only time that you have is now. So manage it well and enjoy every moment. Now is all that you can be certain about.

Bank Cards and Batteries

Most of the people around me comment on my positivity and in all fairness most of the time I am incredibly positive about my life, not because I am trained in the art and science of positivity but because I live as far as possible in the here and now. However sometimes the far flung future pops up and pokes you in the eye and no amount of positive mental attitude can prepare for that.

I was in our local supermarket recently looking to buy two triple A batteries for my television remote control, trouble was I could only buy a packet of four. Plus there was a special offer of one packet for £4.75 or two packets for £5.00. Well let's be honest it made no sense not to buy both packets, despite knowing that two batteries will last for about a year or so. I now had at least four years' worth of remote control batteries.

Brick wall moment – my batteries will last longer than I will. Well even the most positive of people are allowed a meltdown moment, but why did it happen? Simple really, I took my focus from the here and now to four years hence, too painful just don't go there.

Strangely bank cards now have a similar effect. The chances are that their expiry date will be long after mine. Live in the here and now it is the only time available to us, enjoy it, and value it. Ignore the numbers.

Run Over by a Bus?

My younger sister would get quite sniffy with me when I would tell her that it was perfectly possible that she could be run over by a bus before I met my maker. The metaphor being that we never know the minute of our death and it can come quite unexpectedly, as an accident or a heart attack or something similar. My sister though took me quite literally and insisted that she could never be run over by a bus, how could you not notice something so big, noisy, smelly and bright red (where we live), and I had to concede that she probably had a point. That is until recently when one of my clients told me that he had been hit by a bus as a pedestrian, and that he had spent several months in an intensive treatment unit. More importantly he against the odds, survived.

So there you are it is possible to be run over by a bus, seriously though we must live in the here and now. Enjoy every minute that you have because sometimes these buses don't run to time.

The Dead Bag!

I am sure that I must have mentioned my tendency towards control freakery. I was sat around one evening with a group of friends, having a glass or two of wine. We had been discussing strange things that we had gotten up to over the years, my friend commented about my mum and how we had washed her, dressed her, applied her makeup and tonged her hair before we would let the undertaker take her body away.

The discussion then progressed to my son's partner, she had been preparing her bag ready for going in to the hospital for the birth of my grandchild, and she called it the hospital bag. She had put all of the things together for herself and things ready for the new arrival. Suddenly (three glasses of red wine in) I came up with a perfect idea, my 'dead bag' as I explained to my friend if people are going to come and see me then I need to make sure that I look good, and so the idea of the 'dead bag' evolved. The 'dead bag' is to contain matching pillow covers, duvet cover and a nightdress with a perfect matching shade of lip gloss and nail polish.

I haven't actually done it yet but probably will, even if it just gives my friends something to chat about later. I can hear them now, "She really was nuts you know, and she even prepared her own 'dead bag'"

Control freak or what?

The Big C

The Big C is an American television programme where the central character, Cathy has cancer, she lives with cancer and the programme is about her journey, and it is very, very funny. It is also very, very sad.

I was sat watching it last week and wondered about the writer, I haven't researched who wrote the story or the scripts but they are very clever to see the humour in something tragic. What I admire most though is that they treat cancer as a normal part of life, tragic, funny, scary and emotional but a normal natural thing that happens to normal people everywhere.

Think hard and find something funny about your journey, I know that you will have cried buckets and I also need to know that you have laughed too……. Think about the funny things there will be something somewhere

Note to Self

What have I got to giggle and smile about?

The Man in the Supermarket

I consider myself to be incredibly laid back these days, I rarely get angry, and I have never been particularly confrontational. I say what needs to be said and then move on. More and more these days the things that would have made me speak out in the past I now find myself saying or just thinking "it doesn't matter". For example I bought a white suite for my conservatory and before it was a week old my friend had dribbled red wine on the chair and the foot stool. I did not care a jot, we were having fun, and it does not matter. Twenty years ago I might have killed him with my bare hands!

Last Friday I was stood in the kiosk queue at my local super market, I was patiently waiting for a customer service assistant when a gentleman in his mid-fifties, all smartly dressed leapt in front of me and asked the assistant for twenty cigarettes. When I pulled him up he said "sorry love, you don't mind do you, only I haven't got time to wait"

Wow, temporary insanity descended upon me, I grabbed his wrist, snatched his cigarettes and told him in my most stern and serious voice that he could not possibly understand what the phrase "not got time" meant. I explained in detail and quite loudly how 'now' is the most important time to someone living with cancer, and how he had invaded my 'now' and stolen my time, which is precious. I also vociferously highlighted how difficult it is to empathise with a rude arrogant addict who had about as much sensibility as a snail.

When I had completed my rant I handed him back the cigarettes and the other people in the queue clapped, until that moment I had been completely unaware that there was anyone else around me; fortunately I didn't swear!

Oh well, we can all have an off day and we all have things that annoy us. Sometimes we need to be aware of our anger triggers. Being angry can be quite healthy, it just depends on how we do anger. What are your anger triggers and what is the best way to acknowledge your anger. You are possibly angry about your diagnosis, or the impact that it is having on your daily life.

A little while ago I was working with a group of ladies, ladies who had found themselves entangled in the criminal justice system. We were discussing anger and how we do anger, the way that we do anger can be very destructive and get us in to trouble. I asked the group of ladies to call out a four letter word that they associated with anger, well you can probably imagine what words I got and I certainly couldn't print them here. We spent ages looking for the word that I wanted and in the end I had to tell them, the word that I was looking for was NEXT. Sometimes it is safest to acknowledge what makes you angry and if it is something that you cannot control move on. Once again writing things down can help you to put things in to perspective.

Note to Self

Things that make me really angry are

The Bucket List

All of my practical things are now taken care of. I have talked with you about time management, and revealed some of the things that get on my nerves and make me angry as well as some of the things that make me giggle. Fortunately I am still very well, I still work and love my job, and if I am to be honest there isn't much stuff on my list that I still want to do, but I bet that you have? I have a wonderful life. I want to go to my son's wedding and I fancy a trip to Jerusalem but most of all I want to try my best to enjoy every minute as it comes along. I really do focus on living in the here and now, I meditate and use self-hypnosis to help me to relax and remain positive. I love going to the spa and having a massage or spending a spare afternoon in the hydrotherapy pool. So there are plenty of spa visits on my bucket list, in fact every time I have one I add one more.

I also love just sitting in my conservatory reading my books and journaling. I am also an addict! That is I am addicted to watching Frasier repeats, no matter how many times I watch them I still laugh out loud, I need to watch at least one each day to get my fix, I guess that I had enough of Midsomer Murders last year. Laughing in itself is very therapeutic.

Live the life that you love, you really only have today and that applies to everyone, regardless of your state of health, your I.Q or your bank balance. How much happier would we all be if we realised the value of 'now' much earlier in life; it is sad that we have to experience a life threatening disease to realise just how precious each moment is.

TLC Brought me an Angel

Now I don't know whether you believe in angels or not, it doesn't really matter either way, but in my life every now and again something has happened that has made me think that possibly there might be.

I am a champion of the Breakthrough Breast Cancer Touch Look Check campaign (TLC) and I spend quite a lot of my spare time running TLC Road Shows in my local area. What this means is that I set up an exhibition type stand and provide early detection information to the general public, in the vain hope that I might just prevent someone else from walking the road that we are walking now. We all know that early detection gives us a better chance of beating this disease. I talk to ladies of all ages, and sometimes to men, who want to take the information for the important ladies in their lives, and of course to raise awareness that men can contract breast cancer too. One of the things that I have noticed as I have evaluated my efforts is that older ladies, probably seventy plus ladies think that because they have stopped having regular screening that they don't need to check their breasts. Sometimes I find that even ladies in the age group for screening think that they don't need to check their breasts because they have regular mammograms. I try to persuade them otherwise.

One particular day one of my bosom buddies and I were manning a TLC stand in the centre of Warrington in Cheshire and I approached a lady who I guessed was possibly in her mid-sixties, and as sometimes happens she said "I don't need one of those [leaflets]" so I went on to explain to her that regardless of age……… etc. She then explained to me that not only had she been living with breast cancer she had been living with secondary breast cancer for nine years, the first secondaries were discovered in her lungs and she also had bone secondaries which was a relatively new diagnoses. This lady was my angel; I had never met anyone who had survived so long with lung secondaries before. She praised what we were doing, gave me a big hug and went on her way. It is so inspiring to hear someone else's story. That lovely lady made my day.

Letter from a Friend

I guess this lovely letter that I got from one of my dearest friends was a reminder to practice what I preach; I thought that I would share it with you because it contains some great advice.

Dearest Jules

I was doing some research recently when I came across a fantastic programme called "W.I.T.C.H." (Woman In Total Control of Herself). I thought that the principles of the programme might be something you might enjoy and want to try. It's simple to do and with a little time and effort I believe you will see some benefits. It's called P.M.A. (Positive Mental Attitude).

After receiving devastating news about your condition having a positive attitude will enable you to take back control, and enjoy living every day. A positive attitude will serve you and those around you well. Your attitude is something "you can" control. This is a gift to yourself and your family. PMA is certainly no 'Pollyanna' approach, it will however make the difference between a bad day and a good one, and why wouldn't you want every day to be great?

You can accomplish almost anything with PMA; take charge of your day, take control of your thoughts and feelings, they're yours after all. I can guarantee you will feel you are back in 'the driving seat', total control. How great are you? So embrace and celebrate that. Go girl, GO! Throw inhibition to the wind and give it a go, you've nothing to lose, and everything to gain. What are you waiting for? Don't forget a 'high five' or 'yeh' every now and again and that other fantastic therapy, laughter!

Experiences like going to the theatre can be a brilliant night out, a reason to get into your 'glad rags' and local productions are fun and reasonably priced. Perhaps it's time to take up a new hobby but whatever you choose, make sure you have fun and thoroughly enjoy yourself. Remember, a positive mental attitude is the best medicine; it can be taken in excessive amounts, in fact, the more the better! You can't overdose; the more you embrace a positive attitude the easier it will be. Soon it will be second nature and will take no effort at all. Enjoy the new-found freedom your positive attitude will bring, everything is possible, push those boundaries. Remember, there is nothing better than the certainty of knowing that 'you are' in control. Make that change, today make a difference, look forward to tomorrow and the new challenges it has to offer.

Don't really know why I am telling you all this, it was you who wrote the programme. Now you can live the programme and I know that you will inspire many other women along the way.

Your friend Lyn

Last Word about Finances

Do You remember my Nana Mabel? Her surgeon predicted a six month life expectancy for her. She spent her next few months spending every penny of her life savings, doing all of the things that she wanted to do and buying things to make her life more fun. Fabulous stuff!

Nana Mabel lived for twenty-eight years and never forgave her surgeon for living the last twenty seven and a half years in 'poverty'............................. that bus was a long time coming, as I said earlier they don't always run to time.

Finally...

You may not believe this but there are worse things than living with cancer. Perhaps that might be the subject of my next ramble, bye for now and take care of yourself.

Jules

P.S You can find out more about my work at

www.positivewomen.co.uk

www.cmst.co.uk

www.restorativepathways.co.uk

www.ingramcontent.com/pod-product-compliance
Lightning Source LLC
Chambersburg PA
CBHW070856280326
41934CB00008B/1469